Delicious
Nutritious

Every Child's Friend

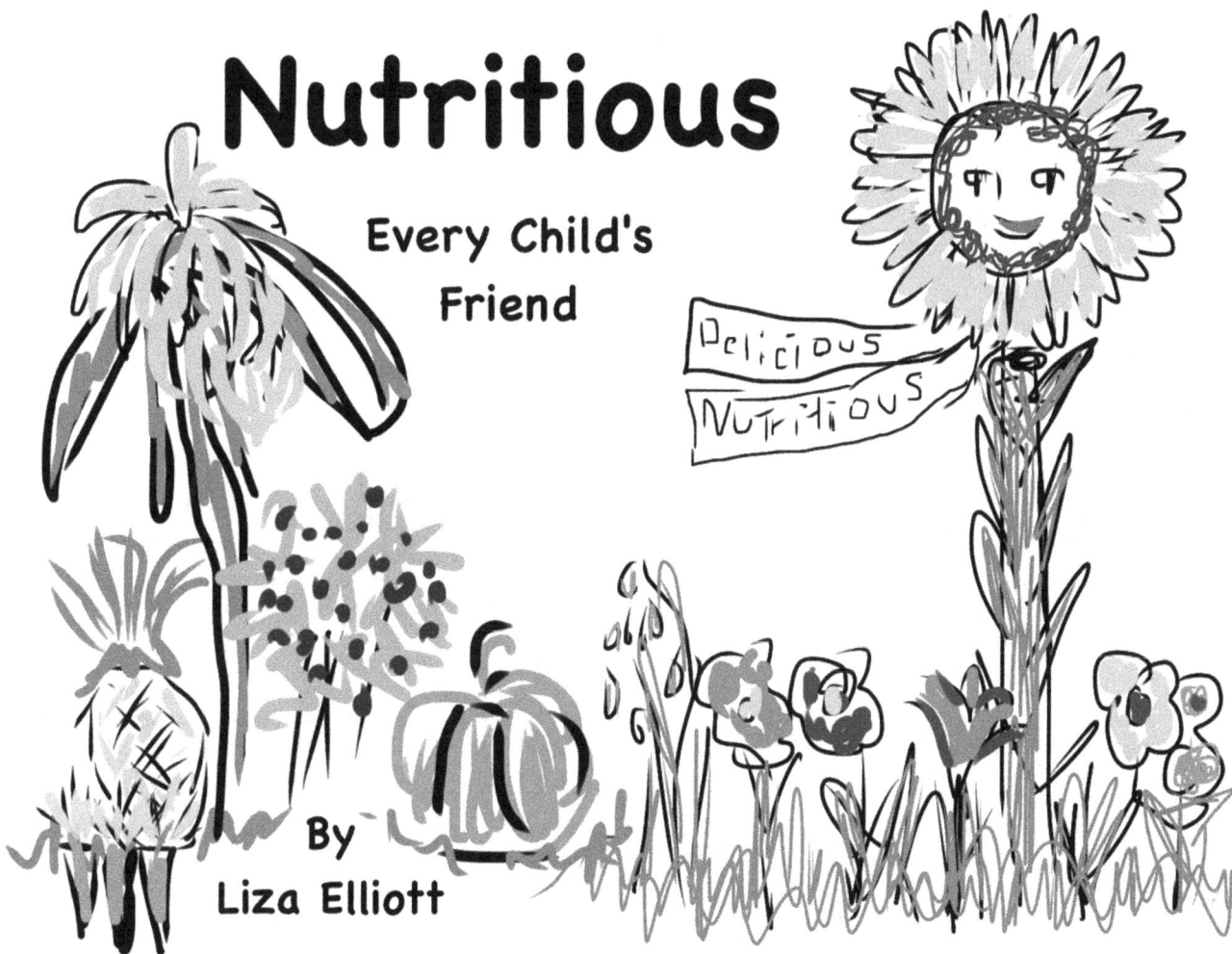

Delicious
Nutritious

By
Liza Elliott

Red Camel Press, Birmingham, Alabama

2014 Red Camel Press

Published by Red Camel Press, Birmingham, AL, USA

ISBN 978-1-937014-06-3

Printed in the United States

www.redcamelpress.com

Library of Congress Control Number: 2014908489
Library of Congress subject headings
Nutrition
Children
Educational
Graphic Art

Book Cover and interior graphic art by Liza Elliott
Nut Free Granola Bar Recipe courtesy of Panther Press, Mountain View, CA.

Special thanks to Tie Hamilton, for her consultation during the development of Delicious Nutritious,
which gave rise to the format of a coloring book.

Special thanks to Kayla White of Kayla White Photography for file set up and book design.

**A portion of proceeds from the sale of this book goes to Delicious Nutritious,
benefiting Children's of Alabama Emergency Department, Birmingham, AL.**

For Anne Warren
whose tireless advocacy for children
inspired the Delicious Nutritious Program

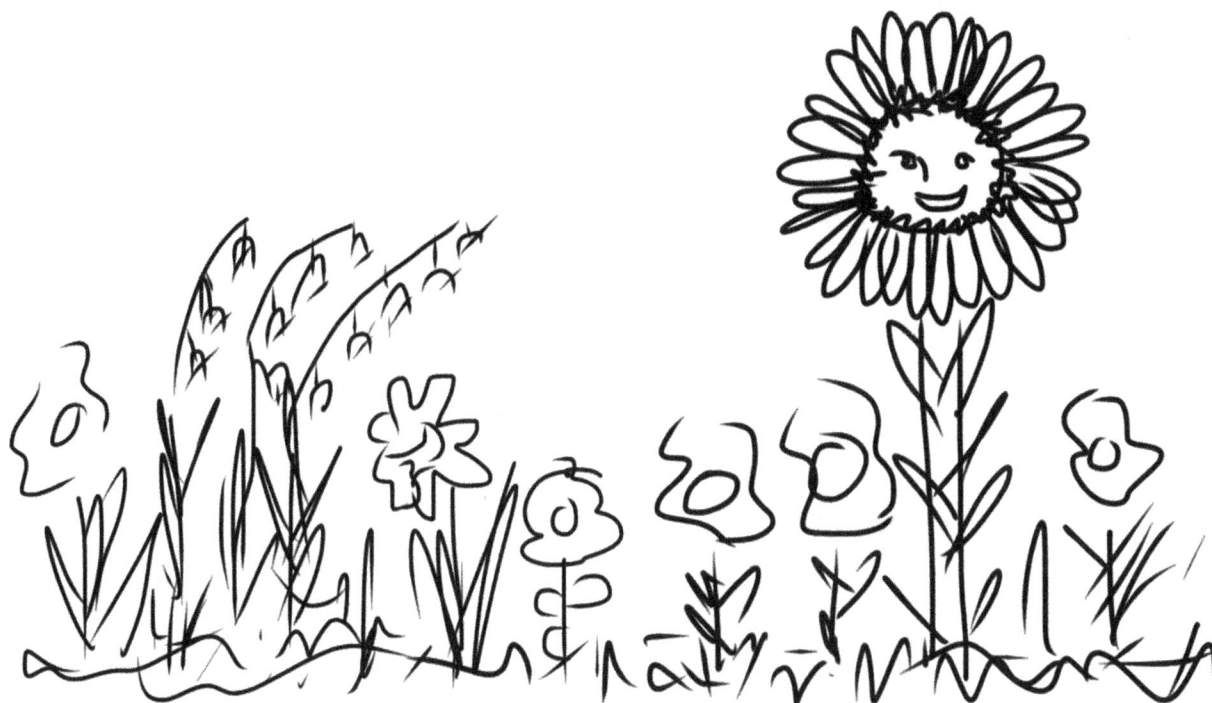

After playing a while, Avery and Jalen

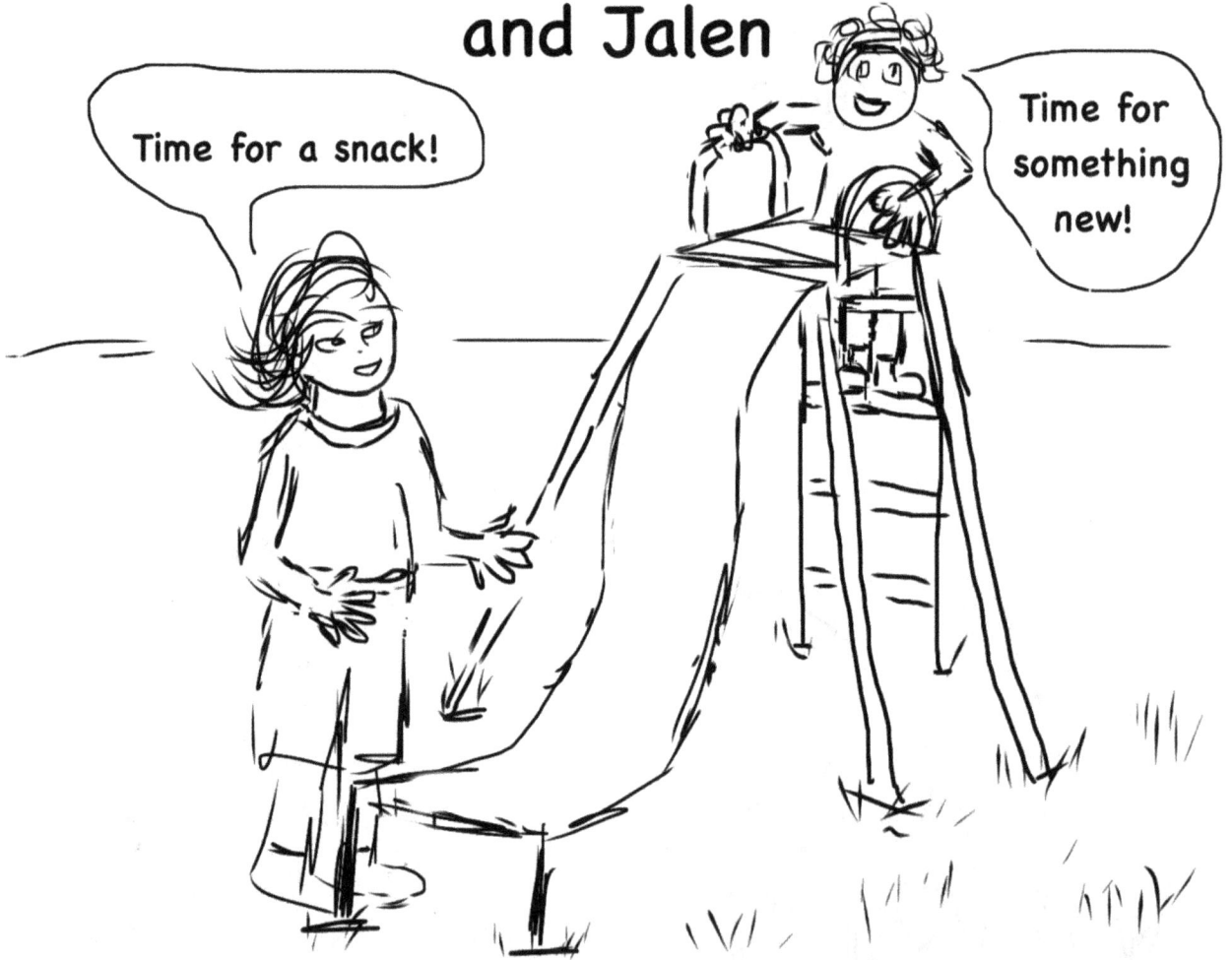

are ready for a snack!

A healthy snack
is what you need!
Help yourself to my
sunflower seeds!

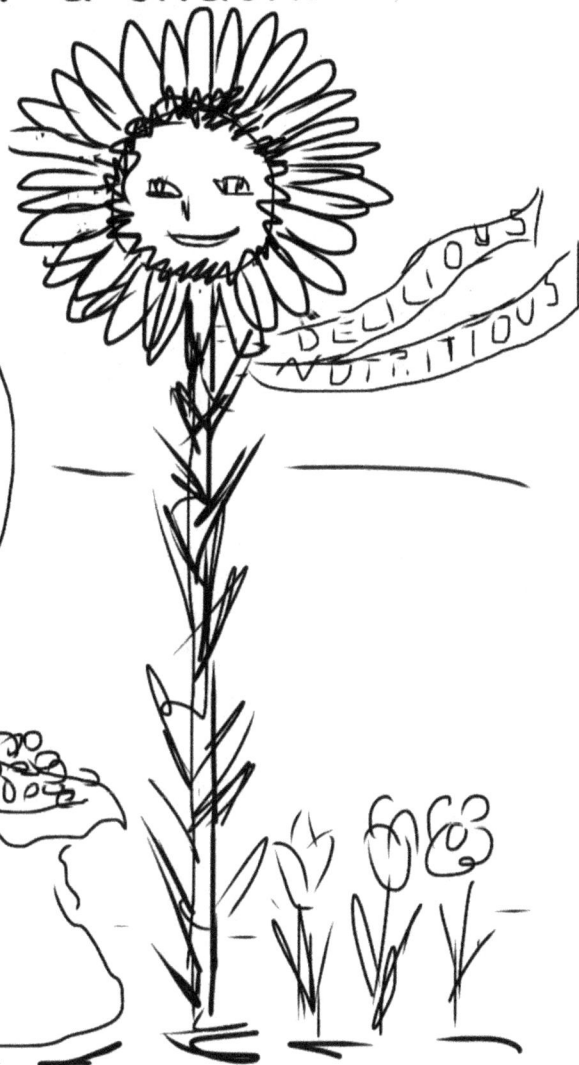

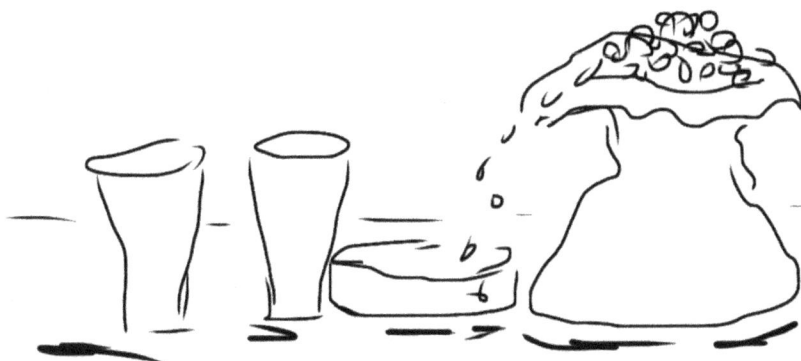

DELICIOUS
NUTRITIOUS

Willow and Violet

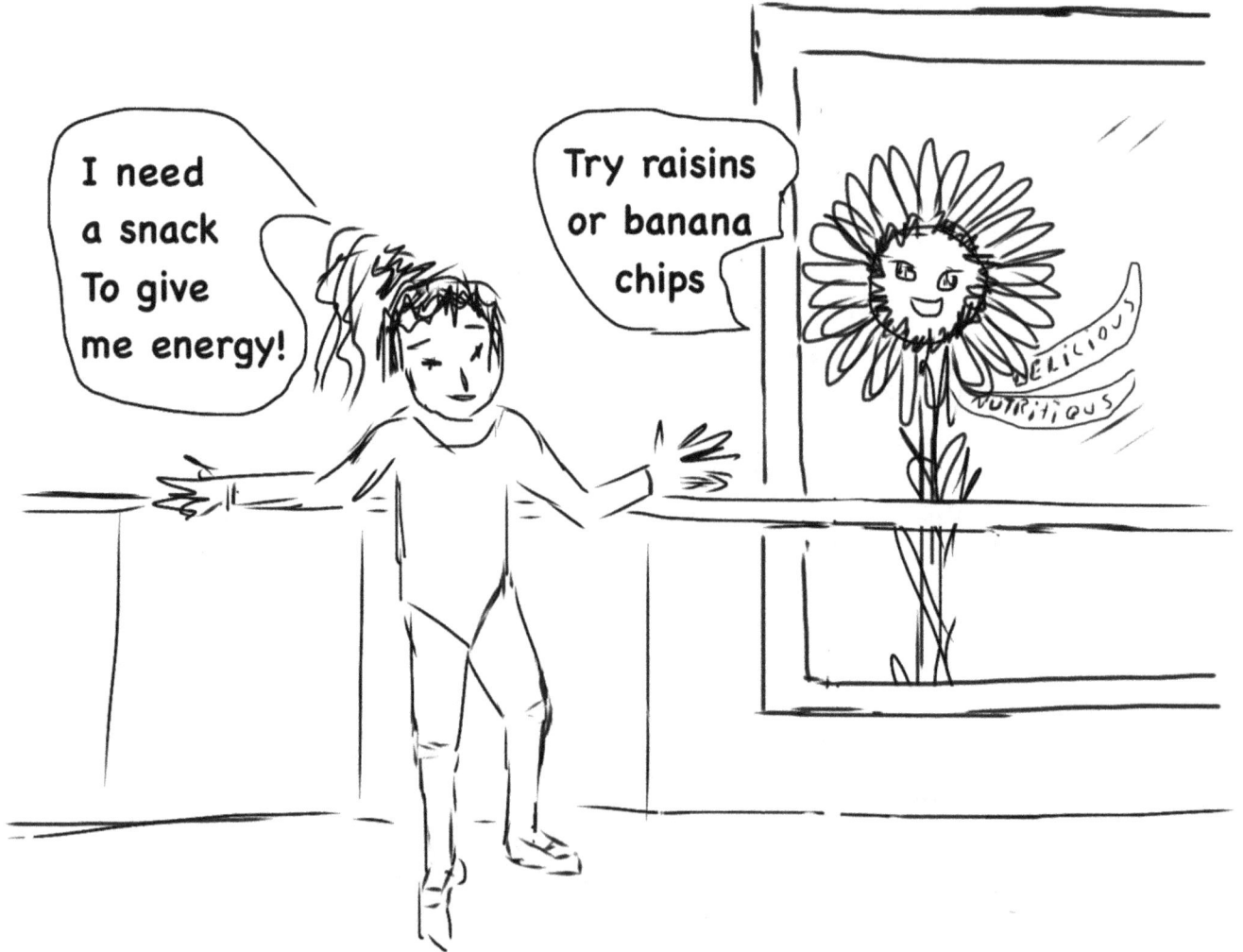

love ballet class.

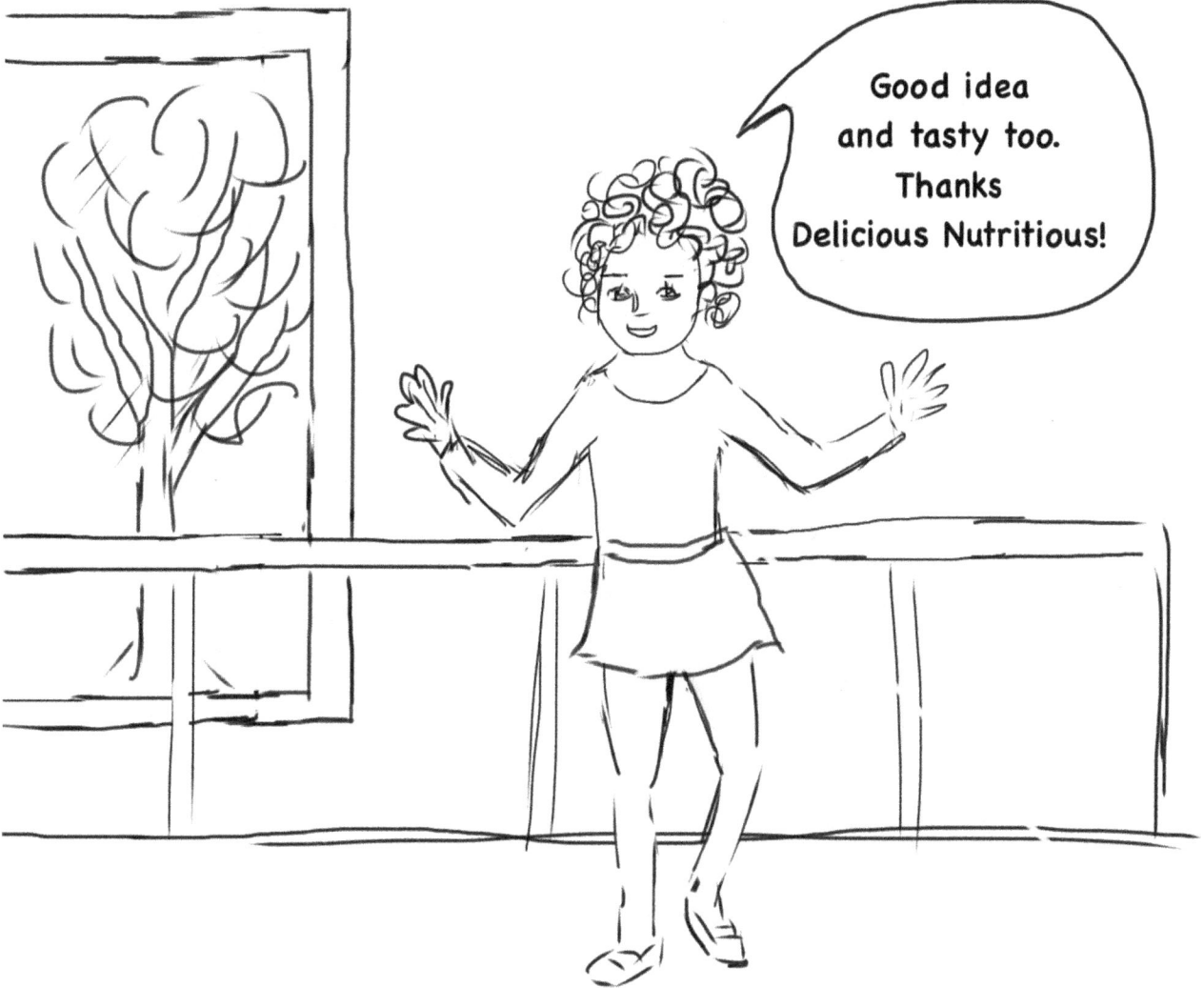

Good idea
and tasty too.
Thanks
Delicious Nutritious!

Eli and José play football

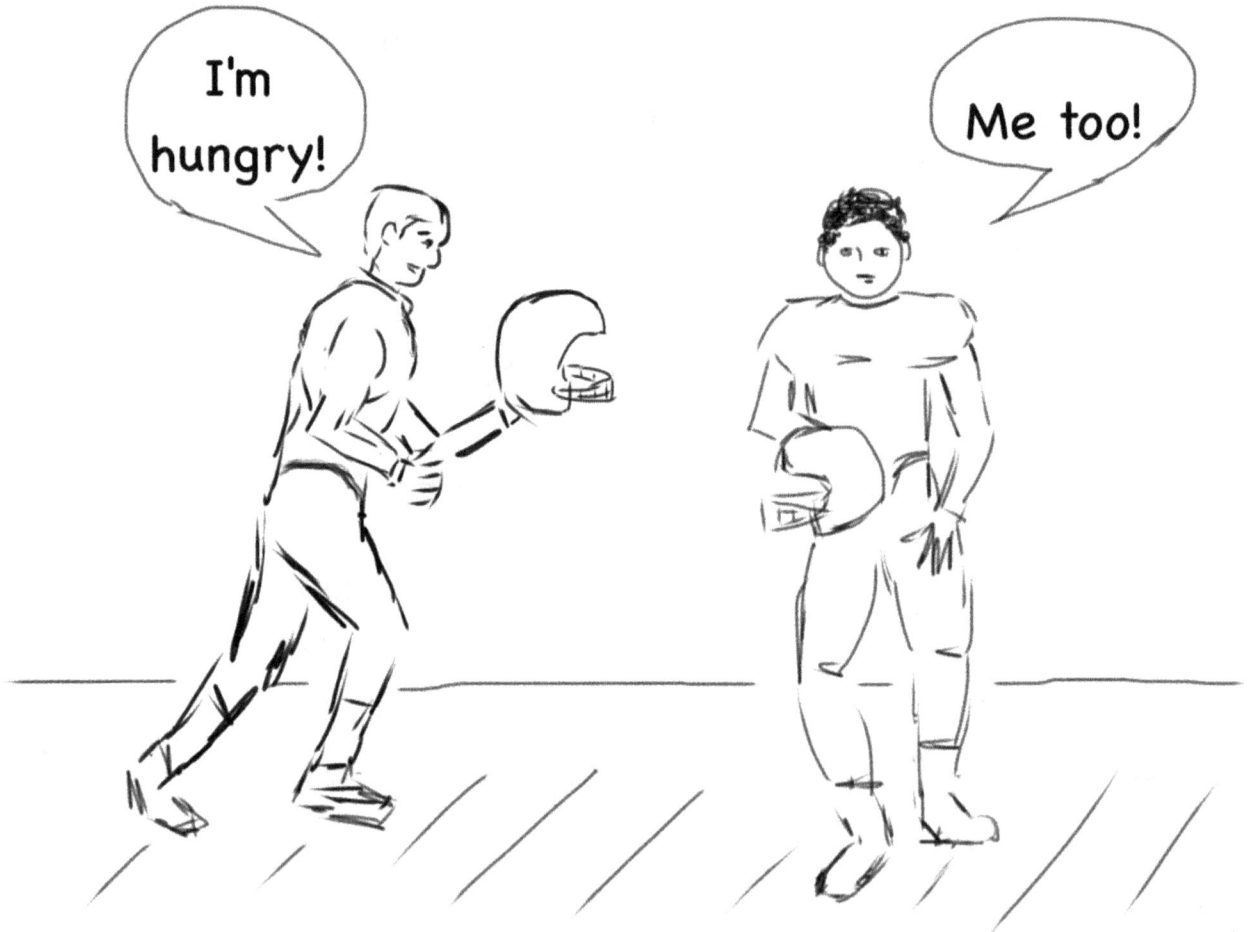

with Ahmad and Chebon.

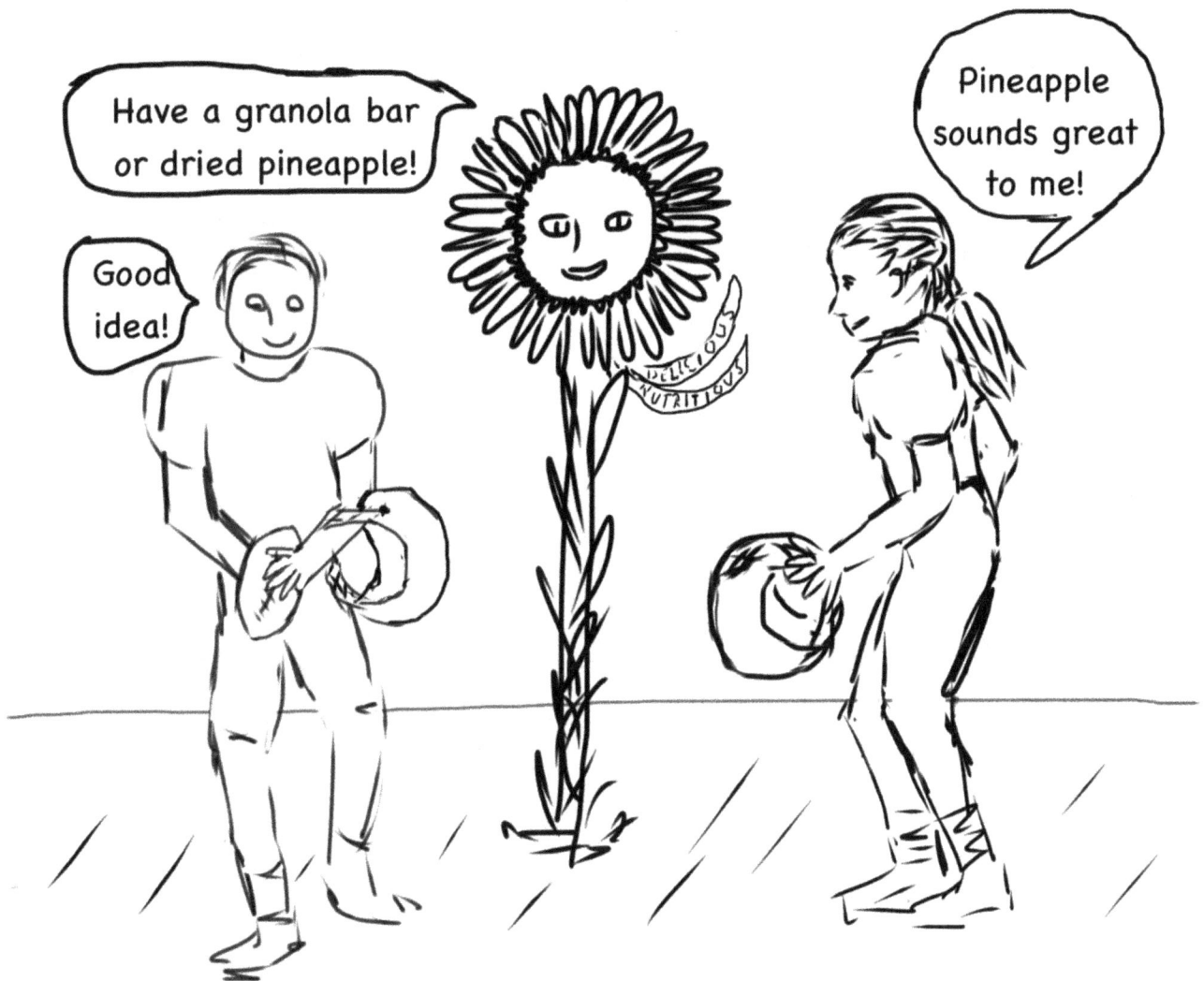

Amira and Sabrina love to run track!

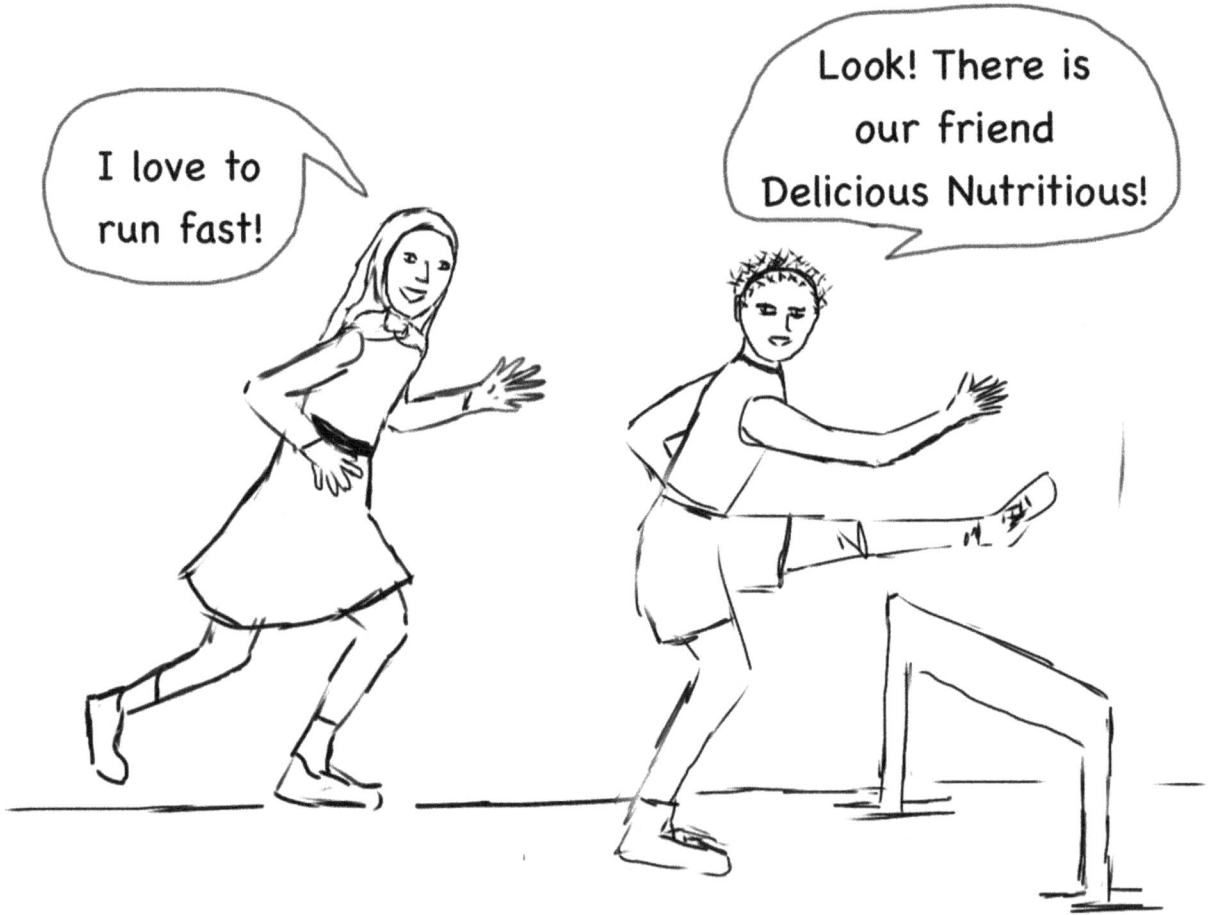

I love to run fast!

Look! There is our friend Delicious Nutritious!

Billy loves basketball!

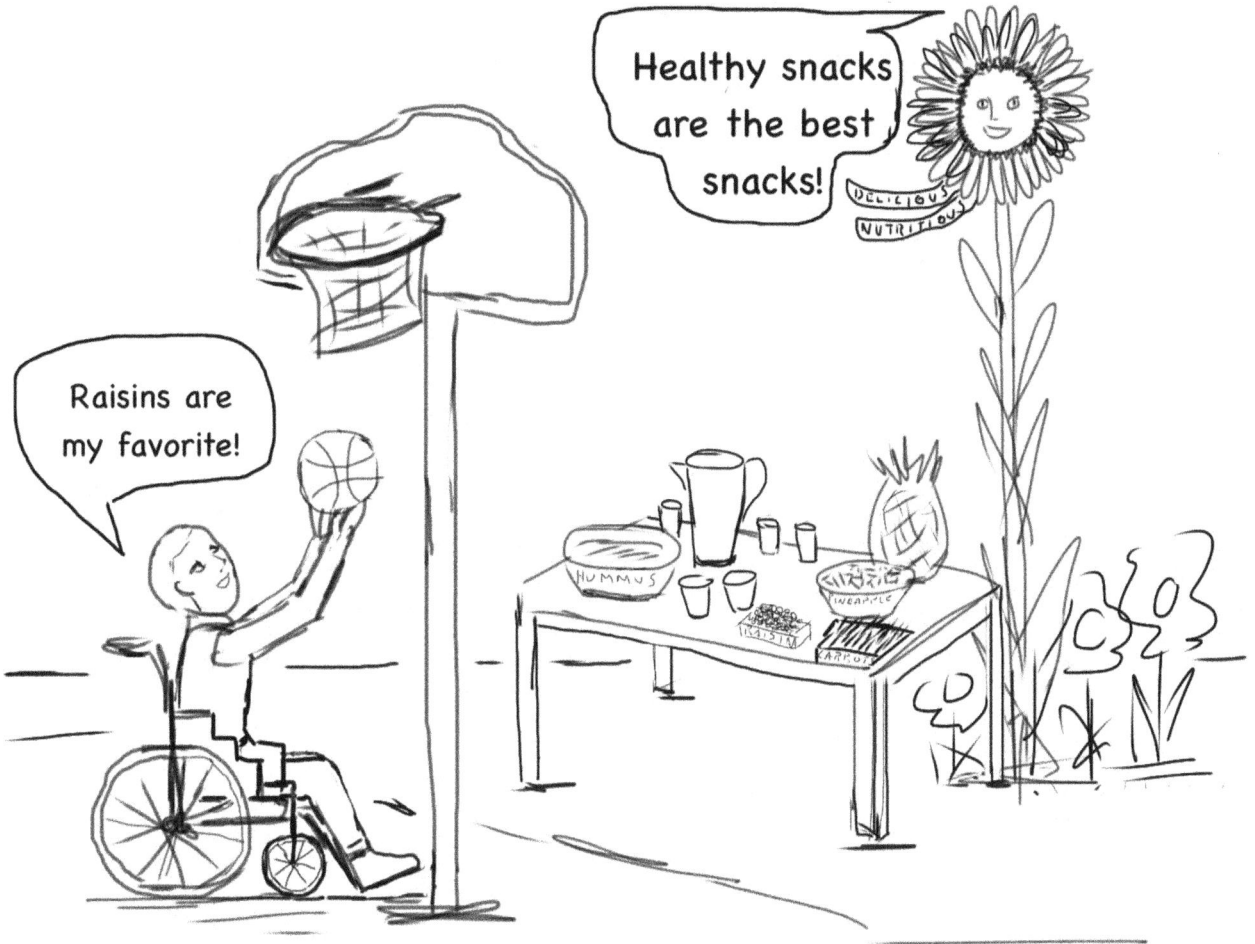

Ravon and Martise love to play soccer!

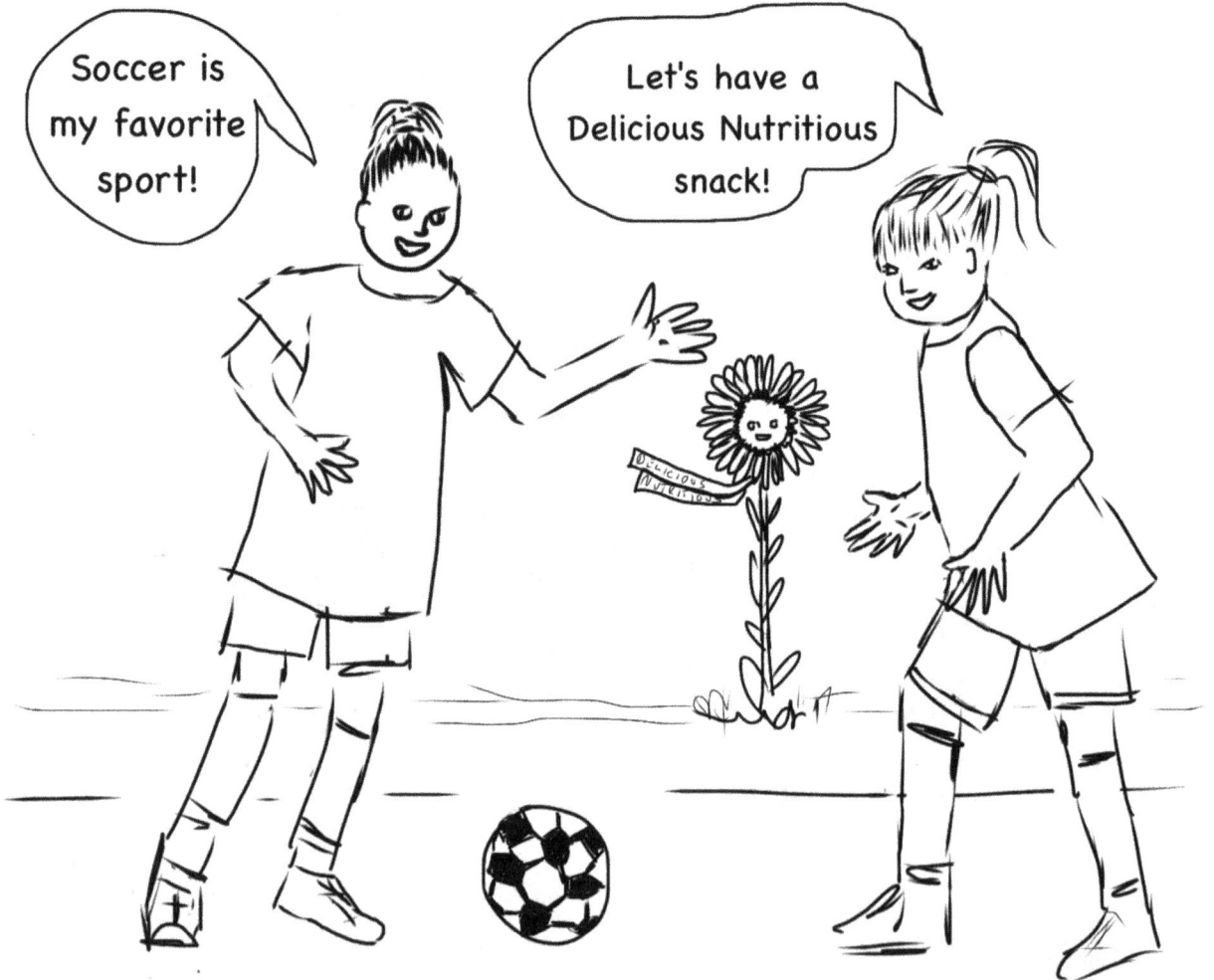

12

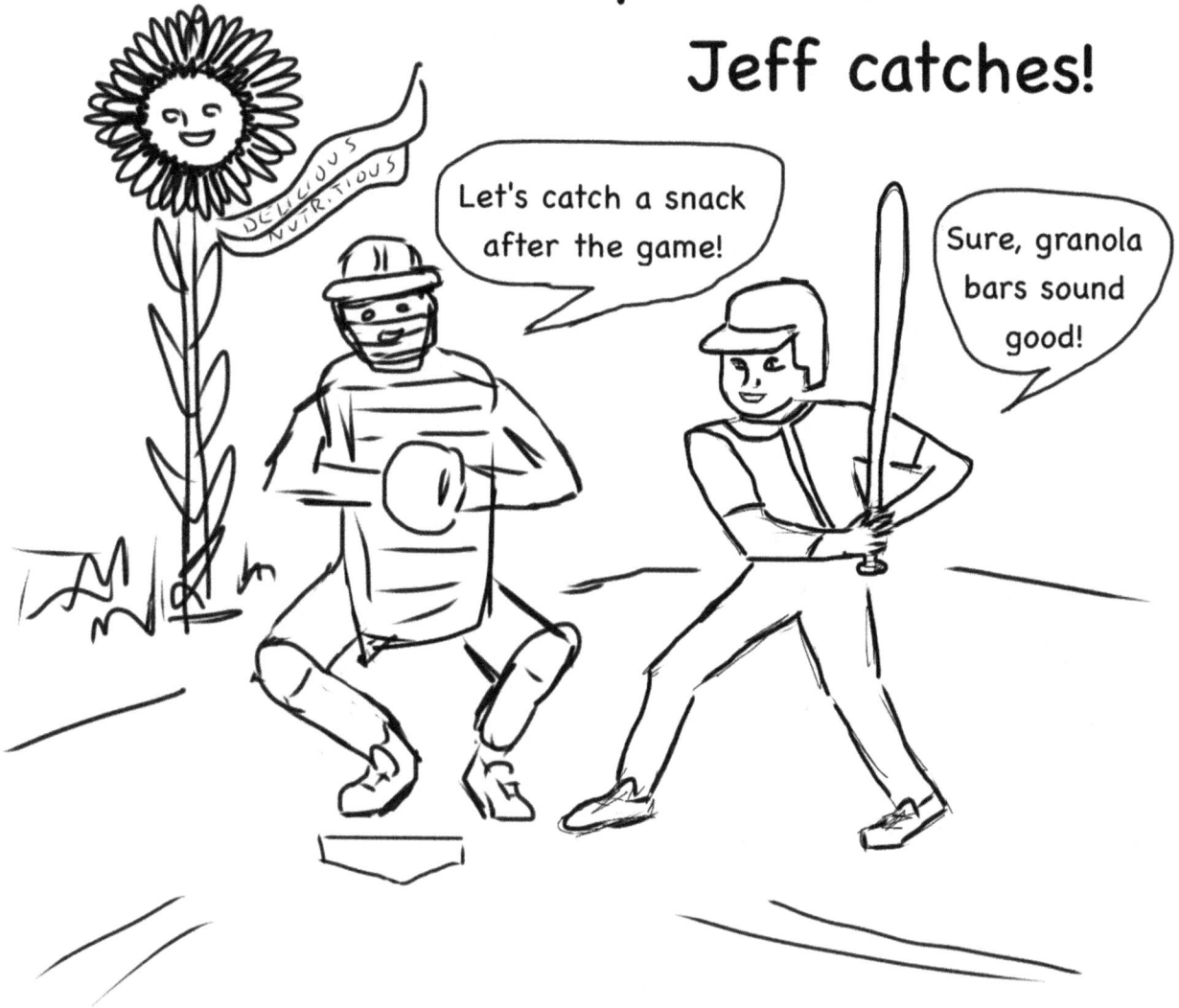

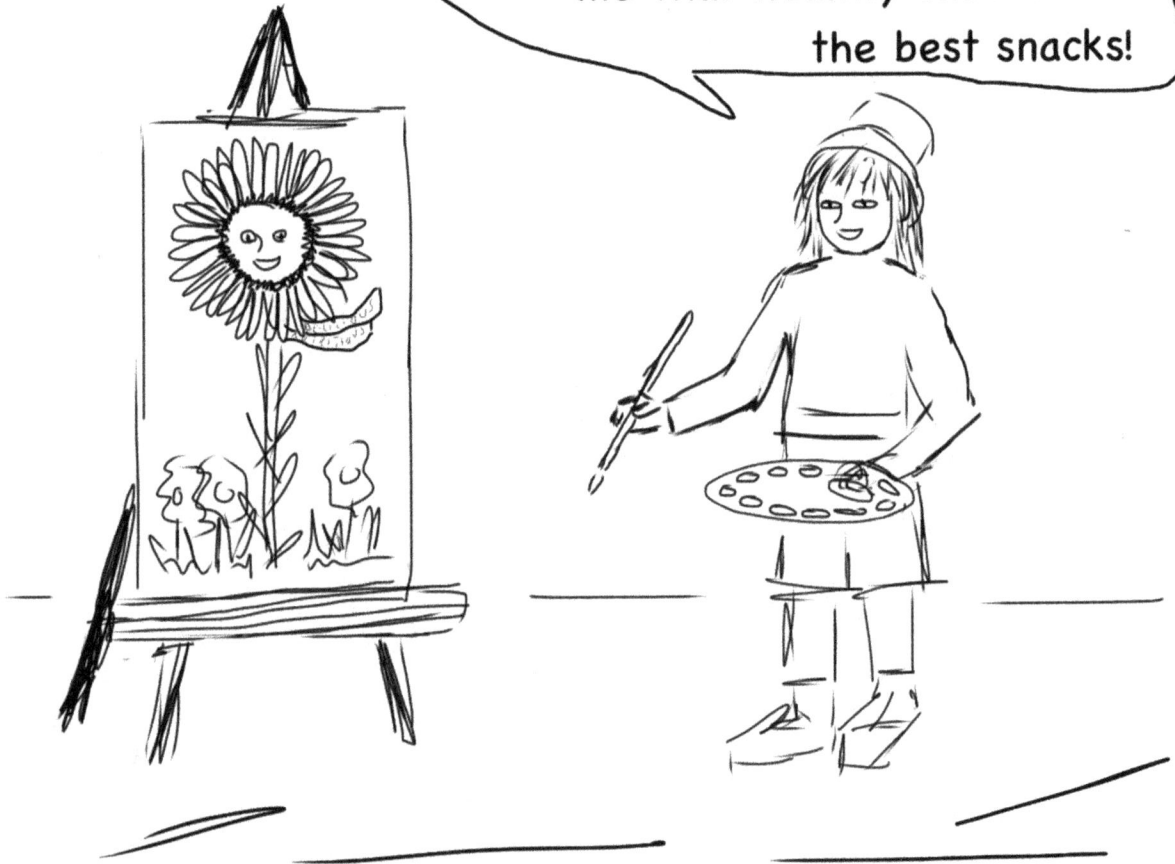

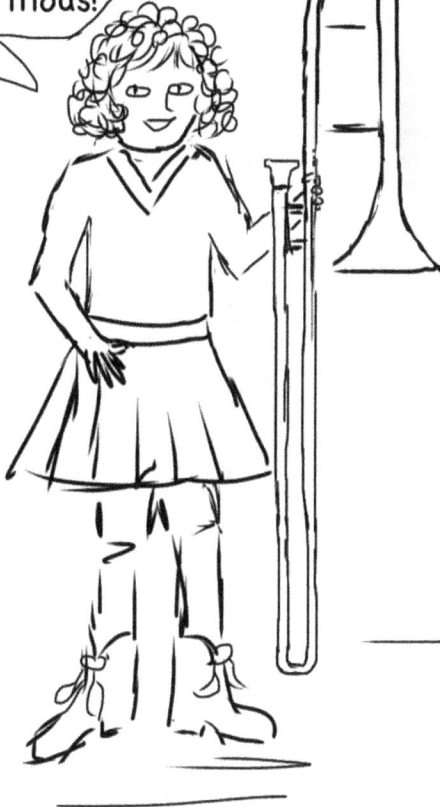

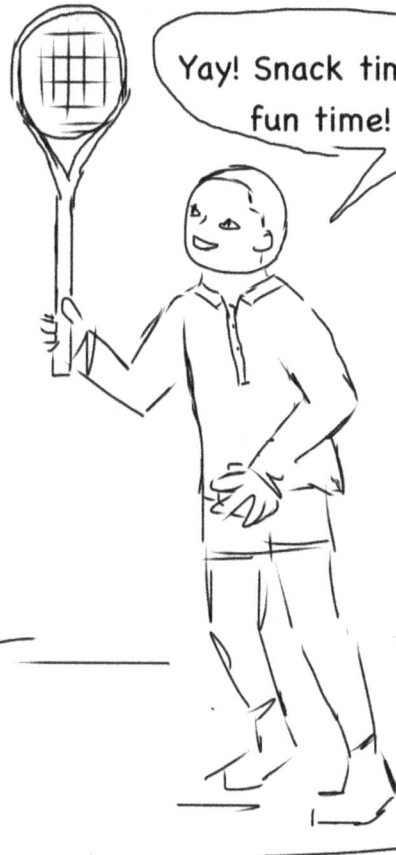

When you want a snack, have a Delicious Nutritious snack!

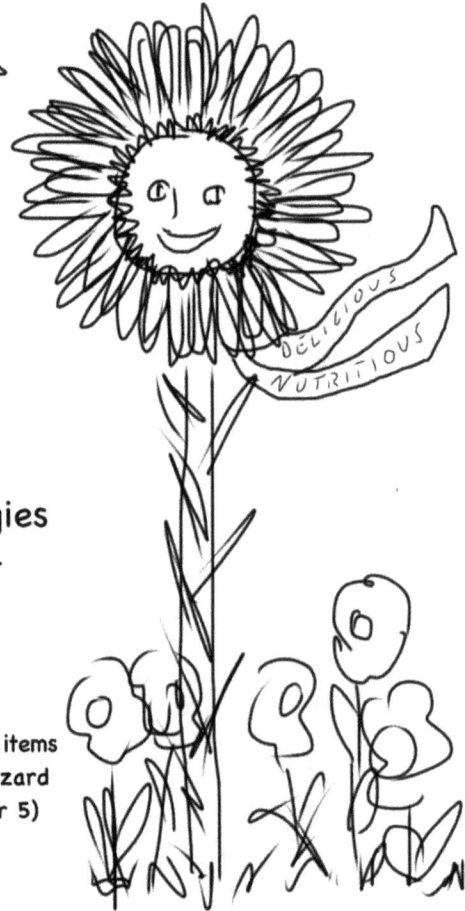

Sunflower seeds
Pumpkin seeds
Nut free granola bars
Dried banana chips
Dried pineapple slices
Assorted dried fruit
Raisins
Yogurt covered raisins
Protein bars

Yogurt
Fresh veggies
Fresh fruit
Cheese

(Remember, small items pose a choking hazard for children under 5)

Nut Free Granola Bars

2 cups oats
1 cup crispy rice cereal
1/2 cup raisins
1/4 cup melted butter

1/2 cup brown sugar
1/4 cup honey
2 teaspoons vanilla extract
1/2 cup mini choc chips

1. Melt butter, add sugar, honey, vanilla
2. Mix together oats, cereal, raisins
3. Mix all ingredients well
4. Spread into baking dish, press chocolate chips on top
5. Chill 45 minutes, cut, and serve

Draw your own
Delicious Nutritious!

Draw your favorite snack!

www.ingramcontent.com/pod-product-compliance
Lightning Source LLC
Chambersburg PA
CBHW051350290326
41933CB00042B/3357